CW00516054

30 ESSENTIAL POOL EXERCISES

FOR SENIORS AND BEGINNERS

A Comprehensive Guide to Low-Impact Fitness, Stress-Free Workouts, easy simple flexibility balance, strength and Healthier Living in the Water

ANGELA CALL

30 Essential Pool Exercises for Seniors and Beginners

A Comprehensive Guide to Low-Impact Fitness, Stress-Free Workouts, Easy Simple Flexibility Strength and Healthier Living in the Water

Angela Call

Copyright © 2023 by Angela Call

All rights reserved. No part of this eBook may be reproduced, distributed, or transmitted in any form or by any means, including photocopying, recording, or other electronic or mechanical methods, without the prior written permission of the author, except in the case of brief quotations embodied in critical reviews and certain other noncommercial uses permitted by copyright law.

This eBook is intended for educational and informational purposes only. The author and publisher are not responsible for any injuries, illnesses, or damages that may result from your use or misuse of the information contained in this eBook. Before beginning any exercise program or making changes to your diet, you should consult with a qualified healthcare professional or fitness expert.

Disclaimer

All trademarks and registered trademarks mentioned in this eBook are the property of their respective owners.

Table of contents

Introduction

Imagine a location where fitness meets enjoyment, where you can begin on a road to a better, happier self without putting your body through a harsh toll. This isn't some far-off fantasy; it's here at your neighbourhood pool.

Welcome to the book "Pool Exercises for Beginners: A Comprehensive Guide to Get Fit in the Water." This eBook is your passport to the revolutionary realm of water exercise. Whether you're a complete novice or seeking to broaden your workout regimen, the pool offers a wealth of chances to improve your health.

We constantly hear about the value of persistence, commitment, and hard effort in the fitness field. But wouldn't it be great if you could achieve your fitness objectives while having fun along the way? Pool workouts provide precisely that: an entrance to a better lifestyle that is not only beneficial but also quite pleasurable.

The pool is a one-of-a-kind setting in which the buoyancy of the water makes every movement an exercise in ease and elegance. It's the ideal spot to start your fitness adventure, especially if you've been put off by the high-impact, high-stress character of many workout routines.

There is a sensation of weightlessness in the water that frees you from the responsibilities of gravity, enabling you to move freely while providing resistance that tones your muscles, burns calories, and supports your body.

I'm delighted to accompany you on this water trip as the author of this guide. My love of pool workouts, as well as my desire to assist people like you reach your fitness goals, inspired me to create this comprehensive resource. With years of fitness coaching expertise and a great love of the water,

From the hidden advantages of aquatic fitness to precise instructions for 30 key pool exercises, the pages that follow provide a wealth of information on pool workouts geared for beginners. This guide will help you reduce weight, gain muscle, enhance flexibility, or simply enjoy the freedom of movement in water.

This eBook, however, offers more than simply exercises. It takes a comprehensive approach to your health, covering everything from nutrition and hydration to keeping motivated and consistent, as well as post-workout recovery and self-care.

The pool is more than simply a location to work out; it's a haven for your physical and emotional health.

Now I'd like to welcome you to plunge in and discover the world of pool workouts, where you may reach your fitness objectives while having a blast. This eBook is your full guide to starting this journey, which promises to make you healthier, fitter, and happier. So, how about we get started?

The pool is ready, and your route to health and enjoyment is only a page away.

The Advantages of Pool Exercises for Beginners

Consider an exercise in which every action is met with resistance, yet your body feels weightless. An exercise that develops your muscles, increases your flexibility, and improves your cardiovascular health while submerged in cold, calming water. Such is the appeal of pool exercises.

Pool exercises have benefits that extend well beyond the bounds of the swimming pool. You may be wondering, "Why should I choose pool exercises over traditional land-based workouts?" you may be thinking." Here are a few strong reasons:

1. Be Gentle on Joints: Have you ever experienced the agony of hurting joints during or after a workout?

Pool workouts give a buoyant haven where the water's buoyancy cushions your joints, making it ideal for people suffering from arthritis, joint discomfort, or other musculoskeletal disorders. If you want to exercise in a way that reduces your chance of injury while also protecting your joints, the pool is the place to go.

2. Low Reward, High Impact: Say goodbye to the hammering and jolting that high-impact land-based activities are notorious for. Pool workouts provide a low-impact option that is especially useful for elders, pregnant women, and those recuperating from an accident. The natural resistance of water tests your muscles without putting unnecessary strain on your body.

3. Better Cardiovascular Health: Swimming or doing aerobic activities in the water makes your heart pounding and your cardiovascular system stronger. Water's distinct qualities provide continuous resistance to every action, resulting in an efficient and effective workout.

4. Increased Flexibility and Balance: The moderate resistance of the water is a fantastic tool for extending your range of motion and enhancing your balance.

It allows you to stretch your muscles, develop your flexibility, and activate your core and stabilizer muscles in ways that traditional land-based workouts cannot.

5. Calorie Burn and Weight Loss: Don't be deceived by the pool's tranquil atmosphere; the calorie-burning potential is tremendous. Pool activities are an excellent alternative for weight reduction since the resistance of the water amplifies your workouts, allowing you to burn calories while relaxing in the pool.

6. Reducing Stress: Water has a relaxing impact on the psyche. Pool workouts not only help to develop your body but also to improve your mental health. The serenity, the rhythm of your strokes.

The rhythm of your strokes, the serenity of your surroundings, and the surge of endorphins from exercise combine to produce a holistic experience that relieves tension and promotes relaxation.

These are just a handful of the numerous benefits of pool exercises. Whether you're a newbie searching for a low-impact fitness regimen or a seasoned athlete trying to spice up your exercises, this eBook is your ticket to reaping these and other advantages.

You'll gain the knowledge, confidence, and inspiration to go on a transforming journey in the chapters that follow. We'll look at various pool workouts that target various muscle groups and appeal to a range of fitness goals. We'll create tailored training routines, discuss the significance of good nutrition and recuperation, and delve into the holistic realm of water-based fitness.

So, if you've ever wished for a workout that would leave you feeling energized, calm, and empowered, now is the time to act. Your sanctuary is the pool, and this eBook is your road map to a healthier, happier self.

As You've taken the first step by accessing this eBook, and I commend your initiative. The trip you're about to embark on has the potential to impact your life in ways you can't even comprehend right now. It's an opportunity to rediscover the excitement of exercise, to rekindle your enthusiasm for life, and to realize your full potential.

As you read on, keep in mind that this isn't just another workout book; it's your personal portal to a world of wellness that's as gentle as it is stimulating. The pool is more than simply water; it is a place of limitless possibilities. It's where your aspirations of health, energy, and change become a reality.

By continuing to read the pages that follow, you are committing to investing in yourself, your health, and the pursuit of a better, healthier life. Your passion and determination are the driving forces behind your achievement, and I am here to be your guide and biggest supporter.

Let me promise you that the route ahead is one of fun, not drudgery, and one of infinite sweat, not of endless gratification. The exercises you'll learn here are more than just water motions; they're steps toward a more vibrant, energetic you.

And as we travel together, you'll realize that the pool is more than simply a place to workout; it's also your refuge for self-discovery and well-being.

The advantages of pool exercises should not be overlooked. You'll find more than a workout in the water; you'll find an oasis of calm, a place where your mind may find rest and your body can be rejuvenated.

Each exercise you learn will give you more confidence by increasing your strength, flexibility, and general fitness.

The road ahead will not be without trials, but with each one, you will discover your inner power. Your fresh talents and developing exercise desire will drive your determination. You'll create a lifetime bond with exercise, converting it from a chore to a delight.

Consider a life in which you enthusiastically anticipate your exercises, and each day brings a new opportunity to become the finest version of yourself. That is the ideal we are pursuing, and you are getting closer to it than you think.

Don't give up now. These pages provide the information, exercises, and inspiration you desire. Continue reading, investigating, and allowing the experience to develop. Your road to fitness, health, and happiness begins here with pool workouts for beginners, and it's sure to be one of the most gratifying adventures of your life.

The Low-impact advantages of water workouts for people of all fitness levels.

Water exercises have been increasingly popular in recent years, and with cause. Water exercises are a low-impact, extremely effective approach to enhance your physical health and general well-being, whether you are a seasoned athlete, recovering from an injury, or just starting your fitness path. In this detailed tutorial, we'll go over the numerous advantages of water exercises and why they're appropriate for people of all fitness levels.

Water Workouts' Low-Impact Characteristics

1. Easy on the Joints: One of the most notable benefits of water exercises is their easy on the joints. Water's buoyancy decreases the impact on your joints, making it a perfect alternative for anyone suffering from joint discomfort, arthritis, or recuperating from injuries.

2. Reduced danger of Injury: There is always a danger of injury with traditional exercises owing to high-impact motions.

The resistance provided by the water creates a safe and regulated environment, lowering the chance of accidents, sprains, and strains.

3. Muscle Strengthening: Water provides natural resistance to your muscles, forcing them to work harder without putting strain on your joints. This strengthens your muscles without placing too much strain on them, making it ideal for people wishing to tone and improve their muscles.

4. Enhanced Flexibility: The buoyancy of water helps you to effortlessly move through a full range of motion. This can lead to increased flexibility, especially for people who have tight or stiff muscles.

Suitable for All Fitness Levels

1. Beginners: Water exercises are an excellent place to start for people new to fitness. The buoyancy of water makes activities more doable, lowering the fear of harm or failure. It's a great way to ease into exercise and gain confidence.

2. Intermediate: Intermediate fitness enthusiasts can benefit from water exercises by including resistance equipment such as water dumbbells and resistance bands. These technologies assist to enhance exercises and allow individuals to advance at their own speed.

3. Advanced: Even seasoned athletes can benefit from water exercises. Deep water advanced exercises may test even the most fit persons, giving a unique and efficient approach to maintain and improve fitness levels.

4. Rehabilitation: Water workouts are frequently advised for rehabilitation purposes. Water exercise's low-impact nature assists people to restore strength and mobility after surgery or injury, speeding up their rehabilitation.

1. Aquatic Aerobics: These entertaining and active courses feature activities like leg lifts, arm workouts, and aerobic routines in the water. They are fantastic for burning calories and enhancing cardiovascular health.

2. Water Walking or Running: Water walking or running in waist-deep water provides a low-impact cardiovascular workout. It's a good alternative for people trying to increase their endurance.

3. Water Yoga: Water yoga combines basic yoga positions with the extra resistance of water. It improves balance, flexibility, and awareness.

4. Aqua Zumba: If you enjoy dancing, Aqua Zumba is the ideal combination of fun and fitness. This high-energy, low-impact exercise incorporates dancing routines and water resistance.

Water workouts provide a variety of low-impact activities ideal for people of all fitness levels. Water exercise routines may help you attain your fitness objectives whether you're a novice or an elite athlete. These workouts not only promote physical health but also give a new and delightful experience.

So, take the plunge and explore the world of water exercises, a varied and inclusive method to improve your entire well-being while protecting your joints and body.

Creating a Healthy and Active Lifestyle

In a society increasingly dominated by sedentary habits and demanding schedules, maintaining a healthy and active lifestyle is an important but frequently elusive objective. We all want bright health, limitless energy, and the vitality to flourish in today's fast-paced environment.

The road to reaching this lifestyle is a personal one, with distinct goals and personal tales. It's a road that takes shape one step at a time via decisions. It all starts with a desire for change, a yearning for energy, and a dedication to self-care that goes beyond just survival.

We'll walk this route together in the following pages, immersing ourselves in the relaxing embrace of the pool to discover the profound beauty of water-based training.

This journey is about more than simply physical transformation; it is about pursuing wellbeing in its entirety. It's about striking a balance that includes not only muscle shaping but also soul nourishment.

Our pursuit of a fit and active lifestyle is inextricably linked to the essence of living fully. It is about relishing each day, appreciating the simple pleasures, and nourishing our bodies and brains. This eBook is more than just a pool exercise handbook; it's the secret to living the life you've always wanted.

But keep in mind that the goal of wellbeing is development, not perfection. It's about allowing oneself to be flawed, to fall and to rise again. It's about developing self-compassion and realizing that even a single step toward your goal is a step ahead.

Let us enter the realm of pool workouts with the understanding that this is a long-term commitment to health and pleasure, not a quick fix.

This adventure is about uncovering your limitless potential, and the water serves as our transformational canvas.

Our goal is to feel better, not simply look better, and to flourish in all aspects of life. It's about finding a way to be the greatest version of yourself, one who is lively, energetic, and exuberantly alive.

This eBook is your guide, friend, and mentor as you begin on a journey toward the lifestyle you've always desired. We'll explore the revitalizing world of pool workouts, discover the joy of moving in the water, and weave fitness into the fabric of your daily life.

Are you ready to embrace the water, your well-being, and a life of permanent health and vitality? Let's go on this road together. It's time to encourage a way of life that appreciates the beauty of being active, and the water is beckoning.

Chapter One: The Fundamentals of Pool Exercises

Welcome to Chapter 1 of your pool workout trip, which focuses on setting the groundwork for your aquatic voyage. In this chapter, we'll get deep into the fundamentals of pool workouts, walking you through the essential principles and setting the stage for your amazing fitness transformation. Let us get started.

Aquatic Oasis

Consider a calm pool, glistening in the warm sunlight, its waters providing a serene refuge from the world's chaotic pace. It's a place where fitness and pleasure collide peacefully, and where you'll begin to alter your notion of exercise. Pool workouts turn the water into your personal oasis of well-being, where you may explore the depths of health and fitness in a calm, buoyant, and eternally refreshing setting.

Understanding the Water Advantage

The special nature of water is at the heart of what makes pool exercises so wonderful. This chapter looks into the science and advantages of exercising in water, highlighting the following major points:

1. Buoyancy: Water's buoyant characteristics lessen the effects of gravity, relieving strain on your joints, ligaments, and bones. This buoyancy is a wonderful gift, especially for people suffering from joint discomfort, arthritis, or movement limits. You'll quickly realize why the pool is a haven for people looking for a mild yet very effective workout.

2. Resistance: While water gives buoyancy, it also provides resistance. This resistance forces your muscles to work harder without the effort and risk associated with land-based training. You'll enjoy the full-body involvement that helps shape your physique and improve your cardiovascular fitness while you do moves in the water.

3. Low impact, high intensity: We'll go into the meaning of "low-impact, high-intensity" workouts and how pool exercises exemplify this notion. Learn how to push your limitations, burn calories, and build muscle while protecting your joints - an equation that makes pool workouts a fitness discovery.

4. Universal Access: Pools are common in many areas and come in a variety of shapes and sizes, ranging from public pools to aquatic facilities and even your own private hideaway. We'll talk about pool accessibility, making it clear that beginning a pool workout journey is accessible to everyone.

5. Holistic Health Advantages: It's not only about physical fitness; pool activities have a wide range of health advantages. You'll enjoy the tranquillity of the water and the mental clarity it provides, as well as stress reduction that goes beyond the pool's boundaries.

6. Endless Possibilities: The variety of pool exercises is unrivaled. As you progress through this eBook, you'll come across a diverse range of motions, routines, and workouts that may be tailored to your personal fitness objectives and tastes. The pool provides something for everyone, whether you want a peaceful water-based yoga session or a calorie-burning aqua aerobic exercise.

In Chapter 1, we laid the groundwork for the rich and wonderful trip that awaits us. Your canvas is the ocean, and your potential is boundless. As you gain expertise and comprehend the unique benefits of pool workouts, you'll find yourself pulled to the calming embrace of the pool, ready to start on a fitness adventure that promises increased health, well-being, and an exceptional enthusiasm for life.

So, let us investigate the enchantment of the aquatic realm, where fitness meets tranquillity, strength meets peace, and well-being meets the water. Dive in and explore the beauty of pool workouts, where training is more than just physical - it's a comprehensive path towards a better, happier you.

Your aquatic experience begins here, in Chapter 1, as we build the groundwork for your metamorphosis with pool workouts.

Why Are Pool Exercises So Effective?

Now that we've defined pool workouts, let's look at why they're so effective:

1. Low-Impact, High-Results: The buoyant nature of water decreases the impact on your joints, which is especially good for people who suffer from joint discomfort or arthritis. This implies you may engage in intense exercises without fear of injuring your body.

2. Unrivaled Versatility: Pool workouts are extremely adaptable. You may modify movements to meet your fitness level and objectives. The pool provides activities for everyone, whether you want to develop your muscles, improve your flexibility, or burn calories.

3. A Cardiovascular Boost: Contrary to popular belief, pool activities may raise your heart rate, offering a fantastic cardiovascular workout. Swimming laps or doing water aerobics might improve your heart and lung health.

4. Mental and Emotional Well-being: The pool's peaceful ambiance is therapeutic as well as comforting. Pool workouts have been shown to alleviate stress, anxiety, and sadness, creating a comprehensive sense of well-being.

Pool workouts are, in essence, a comprehensive answer to your fitness demands.

In this thorough book, we will go further into the art of pool exercises, revealing a treasure trove of routines that appeal to varied fitness levels and aims.

You will not only learn how to do these exercises, but you will also learn how to construct a tailored training plan to fit your individual goals.

So, if you're ready to dive into the low-impact, high-reward realm of pool workouts, let's keep going. We're about to embark on a fitness journey that will be both effective and entertaining.

Prepare to create a splash in your training regimen as we explore the vast and exciting realm of pool exercises for beginners.

The following items may be beneficial for pool exercises

Dive deeply into the world of pool exercises, and it gets even more thrilling when you discover the variety of equipment that may boost your water workouts. While many pool workouts require nothing more than your body and the buoyant water surrounding you, there are tools and equipment available to enhance your experience and maximize the benefits of each stroke, kick, and stretch. In this section, we'll look at the equipment that may be your trustworthy companions on your aquatic voyage, allowing you to get the most out of your pool workouts.

1. Swimsuits:- The cornerstone of any good pool fitness regimen is appropriate swimwear. Choose a swimsuit that allows for ease of movement while yet providing required support.

A one-piece suit or a two-piece with a tight top is an excellent choice for ladies. For maximum comfort, men frequently select swim trunks or jammers.

2. Swim Cap:- A swim hat, while not required for all pool activities, may keep your hair out of your face and minimize resistance in the water, allowing for smoother movements. It's particularly useful if you have long hair.

3. Goggles:- Any water-based activity requires a decent pair of swimming goggles. Goggles shield your eyes from chlorine or saltwater while also providing good sight underwater. For enhanced comfort, look for anti-fog and UV protection goggles.

4. Water Shoes: Water shoes may be useful depending on the surface of the pool.

These shoes improve grip, especially if the pool area is slick, and protect your feet from abrasive pool bottoms.

5. Flotation Devices: Flotation belts and vests are excellent tools for deep-water activities. They assist you in remaining afloat while performing workouts that need you to be suspended in the water. Aqua jogging and deep-water aerobics benefit greatly from flotation devices.

6. Kickboards: Kickboards are an excellent instrument for leg training. They give upper-body support while you focus on kicking and developing your leg muscles.

7. Pull Buoys: Pull buoys are great for isolating the upper body when swimming. They are positioned between your thighs to assist keep your legs floating while you concentrate on arm and core motions.

8. Resistance Bands:- Water-resistant training bands may provide a new dimension of difficulty to your pool exercises. They are adaptable instruments for water-based strength training that help to promote muscular activation.

9. Aqua Dumbbells: Aqua dumbbells are specifically developed for resistance training in the water. They are available in a variety of forms and sizes and are excellent for toning your arms, shoulders, and upper body.

10. Noodles and Water Weights: Pool noodles may be used for a variety of activities, including leg training. Water weights, often known as water dumbbells, are used to provide resistance to upper-body exercises.

11. Underwater Speakers or Music Devices: Consider investing in underwater speakers or waterproof audio gadgets to make your pool exercises even more fun.

Music may stimulate you and make your workouts more enjoyable.

These equipment selections are suitable for a variety of pool activities, ranging from easy water aerobics to rigorous strength training.

The equipment you choose is determined by your personal preferences, fitness objectives, and the precise exercises you intend to incorporate into your regimen.

Remember that, while these equipment can improve your experience, they are not required; you can still get a satisfying and effective exercise utilizing simply the natural resistance of the water.

So, whether you want to maintain it basic or embrace the aquatic devices, your pool workouts will remain a vigor and transformation journey.

You're ready to go on an aquatic voyage that offers strength, flexibility, and a deeper connection with the water if you have the correct equipment.

Chapter Two: Getting Started– Your Introduction to Pool Exercises

So you're standing at the edge of the pool, ready to begin this thrilling voyage of pool exercises. You may experience a burst of excitement, a sense of anticipation, and even a tinge of apprehension. It's completely natural.

We're here to help you every step of the way as you dip your toes into the realm of aquatic fitness, ensuring that your introduction to pool activities is easy, safe, and gratifying.

In this chapter, we'll go over the fundamentals of getting started, laying the groundwork for your aquatic adventure:

1. Selecting the Appropriate Pool or Aquatic Facility: Finding the correct body of water is the first step in delving into the realm of pool exercises. We'll go over the numerous alternatives, including a communal pool, a public aquatic facility, and even your own private hideaway. You'll discover how to choose the place that best meets your needs and tastes.

2. Safety First: As with any physical exercise, your first focus should be safety. We'll go over the most important safety measures you should be aware of before you even get into the water. Understanding how to avoid accidents and how to respond in an emergency is critical to your safety.

3. Getting Accustomed to Water: Being in water might be scary for some newcomers. We'll give you some pointers and exercises to help you feel more at ease and confident in the water. Overcoming your fears is the first step toward enjoying your pool workout regimen.

4. Warming Up: Getting Your Body Ready for Action:** A solid warm-up is essential for avoiding injuries and ensuring that your training is productive. We'll lead you through a series of water-specific warm-up activities to get your body ready for the workouts that follow.

5. Required Equipment: While pool workouts sometimes require little equipment, there are a few important elements that may improve your experience.

We'll cover everything from swimwear and footwear to optional extras like kickboards and resistance bands. You'll also learn how to use these tools properly in order to get the most out of your exercises.

By the end of this chapter, you'll be completely prepared to dive into the realm of pool workouts for the first time.

We'll teach you how to pick the correct setting, protect your safety, feel comfortable in the water, and execute effective warm-ups.
Whether you're entering the pool for the first time or returning after a lengthy absence, these essential concepts will serve as your guide as you embark on your aquatic fitness journey.

Pool workouts are a gateway to a better, happier you, and taking that first step is sometimes the most difficult.

We're here to make your journey as easy as the water around you, guaranteeing that your experience is nothing short of extraordinary.

So, let us go on this exciting journey to better health and well-being through the realm of pool workouts. Dive right in; adventure awaits!

Chapter Three: 30 Essential Pool Exercises for Beginners

After laying the groundwork for your aquatic fitness journey and highlighting the numerous advantages of pool workouts, it's time to get to the meat of this eBook: "30 Essential Pool Exercises for Beginners." This chapter is the treasure box of your water exercises, expertly designed to suit persons of all fitness levels, from the newbie swimmer to the seasoned athlete.

Within the pages that follow, you'll start on a journey that will take you through a variety of activities and routines, each designed to activate your muscles, raise your heart rate, and improve your fitness level.

Whether you're a beginner looking to take your first steps into the world of pool workouts or an experienced swimmer looking to renew and broaden your existing workout routine, this chapter is your ticket to success.

The 30 important pool workouts you're going to see are the product of careful selection, ensuring that they not only target different muscle groups but also offer variants to meet your unique fitness objectives and skills.

These workouts are stepping stones to a healthier, more vibrant self. Let's take a look at what's coming up:

1. Water Walking: We begin with a casual stroll through the pool waters, a basic yet effective workout that will expose you to water resistance and help you improve core strength.

- Step 1: Enter the pool and stand in chest-deep water.

- Step 2: Engage your core and begin walking forward with natural steps.
- Step 3: Continue walking for a defined amount of time, such as 5 minutes.

Muscle Groups: This exercise primarily stimulates your leg muscles and utilizes your core for stability.

Modifications:

- For novices, start in shallow water or with a float belt for assistance.
- For advanced: Increase the walking length or add high knees for extra intensity.

2. Aqua Jogging: For a cardio workout unlike any other, we'll try aqua jogging.

This activity will have you running in the water, mixing the fun of jogging with the healing benefits of water.

- Step 1: Put on a buoyancy belt to keep you floating in deep water.

- Step 2: Begin jogging in place in the water, concentrating on a smooth and controlled stride.
- Step 3: Jog for a specific amount of time (e.g., 10-15 minutes) or combine higher-intensity intervals.

Muscle Groups: Aqua jogging is a full-body workout that targets leg muscles, glutes, the core, and the upper body for balance.

Modifications:

- For novices, begin with a flotation belt at a slower pace.
- For advanced: Increase the effort by running faster or including cross-country skiing exercises.

3 Leg Lifts: You'll soon be working your leg muscles as we work on leg lifts to the side and front, boosting your lower-body strength.

- Step 1: Stand in chest-deep water, hanging on to the pool's edge for balance.

- Step 2: Extend one leg straight out in front of you as far as you can comfortably go, then drop it back down.
- Step 3: Perform 10-15 reps with one leg, then switch to the other.

Muscle Groups: Leg lifts primarily target the leg muscles, particularly the quadriceps and hamstrings.

Modifications:

- Beginners should hold the pool's edge for support and begin with modest leg lifts.
- For more resistance, increase the number of repetitions or utilize ankle weights.

4. Flutter Kicks: This dynamic workout develops your core and legs while simulating swimming action while being securely anchored in the water.

- Step 1: Stand erect in chest-high water, keeping your core engaged for balance.

- Step 2: Keeping your legs straight, alternating raising one leg up and down in a fluttering motion.
- Step 3: Continue for 1-2 minutes.

Muscle Groups: Flutter kicks work the leg muscles, particularly the quadriceps and hip flexors.

Modifications:

For beginners, Hold on to the pool's edge for balance and do gentle flutter kicks.

- For advanced, Increase the pace of the kicks or add a kickboard for more resistance.

5. Wall Push-Ups: We'll take your upper body to new heights with wall push-ups, using the pool's edge as a training partner to improve your arm and chest strength.

- Step 1: Face the pool's edge, placing your hands shoulder-width apart on the edge.

- Step 2: Take a little backward step, keeping your body in a diagonal line.
- Step 3: Bend your elbows to bring your chest closer to the edge, then push back to the starting position.
- Step 4: Perform 10-15 repetitions.

Muscle Groups: Wall push-ups primarily focus the chest, shoulders, and triceps.

Modifications:
- For beginners, start in shallow water or complete the push-ups from a higher place on the edge.
- For advanced: Increase the amount of repetitions or attempt slanted push-ups for increased challenge.

6. Pool Noodle Workouts: A pool noodle, a basic yet versatile item, will become your ally as we explore numerous workouts that improve your flexibility, balance, and strength. You'll learn how to utilize the noodle to support your body and enhance resistance, making your exercises more effective and pleasurable.

- Step 1: Place a pool noodle beneath the water's surface with both hands.
- Step 2: Push the noodle down to create resistance, then draw it back up.
- Step 3: Perform 10-15 repetitions.

Muscle Groups: This workout works the upper body, specifically the shoulders, arms, and back.

Modifications:

- For beginners, start with a lighter or smaller noodle to lessen resistance.
- For more resistance, choose a longer or thicker noodle.

7. Water Aerobics: Ready to join an energizing group workout? We'll introduce you to the energizing world of water aerobics, which combines the support of water with the advantages of aerobic exercise.

You'll be surprised how much fun it is to keep active with others in the pool.

- Step 1: If your pool has a water aerobics class, sign up for one or follow the instructions of an instructor.
- Step 2: Follow the instructor's lead and participate in a range of activities including leg lifts, arm circles, and running.
- Step 3: Attend the class for the allotted time, which is generally 30-45 minutes.

Water aerobics is a full-body workout that targets the legs, arms, core, and cardiovascular conditioning.

Modifications:

- For beginners, begin with low-impact versions and progress at your own speed.
- For advanced: Increase the intensity or explore deep water aerobics for a tougher challenge.

8. Knee-to-Chest Stretch: The knee-to-chest stretch is a good introduction to the world of moderate stretching exercises. Your lower back and hip flexibility will thank you for this pleasant and calming practice.

- Step 1: Stand with your arms outstretched for balance in chest-deep water.
- Step 2: To get a light stretch, bring one knee up to your chest and hold it there with both hands.
- Step 3: maintain the stretch for 15 to 30 seconds before moving on to the other leg.

Muscle Groups: The lower back and hip flexors are the main areas of focus of this stretch.

Modifications:

- Beginners should use the edge of the pool as additional support while executing the stretch.
- Advanced: To improve balance and attention, lengthen the stretch and do it while closing your eyes.

9. Water Cycling: You'll be excited to learn about water cycling if you enjoy riding. This low-impact exercise is ideal for improving your cardiovascular fitness and strengthening your legs because it is supported by water.

- Step 1: If a water bike or pedals are available, secure your feet in them.
- The second step is to start peddling in the water to mimic riding.
- Step 3: Cycle for a predetermined amount of time, like 15-20 minutes.

Muscle groups: The leg muscles, such as the quadriceps, hamstrings, and calf muscles, are the ones that water cycling predominantly targets.

- For those who are just starting out, slow things down to a speed that seems natural.
- Advanced: Increase the resistance or the pace, or think about using interval training for a harder exercise.

10. Water Yoga: Immerse yourself in the serene realm of water yoga, where the calming effects of water help you to improve your yoga practice. We'll look at positions that improve balance, flexibility, and relaxation.

- Step 1: Either practice water yoga on your own or enroll in a class taught by a professional.
- Step 2: While submerged in the water, practice yoga postures including the downward dog, tree position, and warrior pose.

- Step 3: Spend 20 to 30 minutes concentrating on balance and attentive movement.

Muscle Groups: Depending on the positions used, water yoga improves balance, flexibility, and targets certain muscle areas.

Modifications:

- Beginners should start with simple positions and provide extra support with a pool noodle or flotation device.
- For those who are more experienced: Try harder yoga positions or extend the time you spend practicing water yoga.

11. Standing Bicycle Kicks: This workout works your legs hard and raises your heart rate by simulating the motion of riding a bicycle while standing in water.

- Step 1: Stand in waist-deep water while stabilizing yourself with your core.

- Step 2: Start simulating the motion of riding a bicycle by raising one knee at a time.
- Step 3. Cycle for one to two minutes.

Muscle Groups: Standing bicycle kicks focus mostly on your leg muscles, such as the quadriceps and hamstrings.

- For novices, adjust the rate and water depth to start off more slowly.
- For those who are more experienced: Quicken the cycle and add modifications like high knees.

12. Water plank: balance can improve your core stability and strength. They'll try to keep your body stable while you're floating in the water.

- Step 1: Place your hands shoulder-width apart on the side of the pool while you stand in chest-deep water.

- Step 2: Maintain a tight core as you extend your body in a straight line from head to heels.
- Step 3: is to maintain the plank posture for 20 to 30 seconds.

Muscles: The core muscles are the ones that water planks primarily target.

modification

- Beginners should start with a shorter plank time and a shallower water level as modifications.
- For those who are more experienced, lengthen the exercise or, for an additional challenge, add leg lifts or knee tucks.

13. Aqua Lunges: While providing an excellent lower-body exercise, aqua lunges also put your balance and stability to the test.

- Step 1: Stand in chest-deep water and tighten your abdominal muscles for stability.

- Step 2: Recreate the action of cross-country skiing by gliding one leg backward and one leg forward alternately.
- Step 3. Skip for two to three minutes.

Muscle Groups: Cross-country skiing in water works the muscles in your legs, arms, and shoulders, as well as your upper body.

Modifications:

- For newcomers: Perform the exercise in shallower water at first and at a slower rate.
- For more experienced skiers: Quicken your pace or use weights like water dumbbells for resistance.
- Water planks are a strenuous workout that's gentle on your joints and can help you strengthen your core.
- Step 1: Stand in chest-deep water while stabilizing yourself with your core.

- Step 2: In position, sprint as quickly as you can while pumping your arms to increase the pace.
- Step 3. Run for 30 to 60 seconds.

Muscle groups: Water sprints work the legs, especially the quadriceps, and are a great cardiovascular exercise.

Modifications:

- Beginners should begin with shorter sprint intervals and at a slower pace.
- Advanced: Extend the sprint time or test your balance by using a flotation belt.

15. Cross-Country Skiing: Before you know it, you'll be gliding through the water in a manner that resembles cross-country skiing, which offers a whole body exercise and significant cardiovascular advantages.

- Step 1: Engage your core while standing in chest-deep water.

- Step 2: To go ahead, alternately kick your legs in the water to simulate swimming.
- Step 3. Kick for one to two minutes.

Muscle Groups: Leg muscles, particularly the quadriceps and calf muscles, are used during water kicks.

Modifications:

- Beginners should start out gently kicking and use a flotation device to keep their balance.
- For more experienced kickers, increase the speed or add ankle weights for more resistance.

16. Water sprints: Water sprints are a great option for an aggressive cardio workout. They'll make your muscles and heart beat quickly.

- Step 1: Stand erect in water that is chest-deep.

- Step 2: Start kicking your legs and making circular motions with your hands to start treading water.
- Step 3: Walk for two to three minutes.

Muscle groups: Treadwater is a great all-around exercise that works your arms, legs, and core while enhancing both your cardio and strength.

Modifications:

- Use a float belt or noodle to help with treading and keep a slower speed if you're a novice.
- For those who are more experienced, lengthen the exercise or add eggbeater or sculling kicks for more force.

17. Water kicks, in which you move yourself forward by kicking your legs in the water, will increase your leg strength and cardiovascular fitness.

- Step 1: Place one foot on the edge of the pool and stand facing it.
- Step 2: Lift your body up till your leg is straight by pushing through the foot on the edge.
- Step 3: Retract your body downward.
- Step 4: Complete 10 to 15 repetitions on one leg before switching to the other.

Muscles: Poolside step-ups mainly work the glutes and quadriceps muscles in the legs.

Modification:

- For those just starting out, adjust by using a step that is lower or a pool area that is shallower.
- For more difficult exercises, up the repetition count or add ankle weights for more resistance.

18. Tread water: Treading water is not just a survival skill, but it's also a great method to exercise your whole body and build endurance.

- Step 1: Stand in chest-deep water while maintaining a tight core.
- Step 2: Jump on one leg, raise the other knee, and then change your leg positions.
- Step 3. Hop for a few minutes.

Muscles: Water hops are a dynamic workout that tests your balance while working your legs, especially the quadriceps and calf muscles.

Modification:

- Beginners could modify by doing smaller hops and using a float belt as support.
- For more experienced players, increase the hopping intensity by increasing the hopping speed or height.

19. Poolside Step-Ups: Step-ups, which focus on your leg muscles and increase your heart rate, may be done near the side of the pool.

- Step 1: Stand in chest-deep water while stabilizing yourself with your core.

- Step 2: In your hands, hold a little medicine ball or another buoyant item.
- Step 3: Walk on water, raising the ball off the water with your arms.
- Step 4: Walk for two to three minutes.

Muscle Groups: This exercise gives a thorough workout to your arms, legs, core, and other upper and lower body muscles.

Modification:

- Beginners should start with a lighter or smaller buoyant item and move more slowly.
- Advanced: Increase the weight of the medicine ball or increase the time spent treading for more resistance.

20. Water Hops: This exciting and difficult workout improves your leg strength and coordination by combining hopping and jumping in the water.

- Step 1: Stand in chest-deep water while keeping your balance by contracting your abs.
- Step 2: Carry out a series of balancing drills include raising one leg out to the side, standing on one leg, and other tree stance variants.
- Step 3: Concentrate for a minute or two on stability and balance.

Exercises that increase balance in the water focus on your legs and core while also enhancing stability and coordination in general.

Modifications:

- For novices, start with easy balancing drills and support yourself with a flotation device or noodle.
- For those who are more advanced: Increase the complexity and length of your balance postures and practice sessions.

21. Water Toning: Dive into a full-body toning routine that incorporates a range of movements, such as leg lifts and arm circles, all while immersed in the water.

- Step 1: Stand in chest-deep water, engaging your core for balance.
- Step 2: Perform a series of movements, including leg lifts, arm circles, and side leg lifts, to target various muscle groups.
- Step 3: Continue for 2-3 minutes.

Muscle Groups: Water toning exercises offer a full-body workout, targeting legs, arms, core, and enhancing cardiovascular fitness.

Modifications:

- For beginners: Start with slower movements and use a flotation device for support.
- For advanced: Increase the pace, add resistance with water dumbbells, or incorporate more complex movements.

22. Water Ball Exercises: A beach ball can be your workout partner in the pool. These exercises add an element of fun while improving balance and strength.

- Step 1: Stand in chest-deep water, holding a beach ball with both hands.
- Step 2: Perform a variety of exercises, including chest presses, rotations, and passes, with the beach ball.
- Step 3: Continue for 2-3 minutes.

Muscle Groups: Water ball exercises engage your upper body muscles, focusing on the arms, chest, and shoulders, while also promoting core strength.

Modifications:

- For beginners: Use a lightweight or smaller ball and maintain a slower pace.
- For advanced: Use a larger, heavier ball, or increase the intensity by incorporating more challenging movements.

23. Noodle Ab Crunches: Work your core muscles with the help of a pool noodle, making ab crunches both enjoyable and effective.

- Step 1: Sit on the edge of the pool with your hands on the pool's edge behind you, fingers pointing forward.
- Step 2: Lift your body off the edge and bend your elbows, lowering your body toward the water.
- Step 3: Push your body back up to the starting position.
- Step 4: Perform 10-15 reps.

Muscle Groups: Poolside tricep dips primarily target the triceps, shoulders, and chest.

Modifications:

- For beginners: Start with a shallower pool area, or use a flotation device for support.

- For advanced: Increase the number of repetitions or use a lower platform to deepen the dip.

24. Poolside Tricep Dips: The edge of the pool is an excellent support for tricep dips, strengthening your arm muscles.

- Step 1: Stand in chest-deep water, engaging your core.
- Step 2: Extend your arms straight out to the sides and create resistance by moving your arms in small, controlled circles.
- Step 3: Perform circles in both directions for 1-2 minutes each.

Muscle Groups: Water resistance arm circles primarily target your arm and shoulder muscles.

Modifications:

- For beginners: Start with smaller circles and maintain a slower pace.

- For advanced: Increase the size of the circles and add resistance with water dumbbells or resistance bands.

25. Water Resistance Arm Circles: In this exercise, we'll focus on your upper body by using water resistance to target your arm muscles.

- Step 1: Stand in chest-deep water, engaging your core.
- Step 2: Extend your arms straight out to the sides and create resistance by moving your arms in small, controlled circles.
- Step 3: Perform circles in both directions for 1-2 minutes each.

Muscle Groups: Water resistance arm circles primarily target your arm and shoulder muscles.

Modifications:

- For beginners: Start with smaller circles and maintain a slower pace.

- For advanced: Increase the size of the circles and add resistance with water dumbbells or resistance bands.

26. Water Bicycle Crunches: Engage your core with bicycle crunches in the water, a fantastic exercise for toning your abdominal muscles.

- Step 1: Sit on the edge of the pool with your legs in the water.
- Step 2: Engage your core and perform bicycle crunches by bringing one knee toward your chest while simultaneously twisting to touch your opposite elbow to that knee.
- Step 3: Perform 10-15 reps on each side.

Muscle Groups: Water bicycle crunches engage your core and oblique muscles.

Modifications:

- For beginners: Start with smaller movements and use a flotation device for support.
- For advanced: Increase the number of repetitions or extend your legs further during the crunches.

27. Water Weightlifting: Discover how you can incorporate water dumbbells or resistance bands into your aquatic workouts to increase resistance and enhance strength.

- Step 1: Stand in chest-deep water, holding water dumbbells or resistance bands in your hands.
- Step 2: Perform a series of exercises, such as bicep curls, lateral raises, and tricep extensions, with the added resistance.
- Step 3: Continue for 2-3 minutes.

Muscle Groups: Water weightlifting targets your upper body muscles, including the arms, shoulders, and chest.

Modifications:

- For beginners: Use lighter resistance or start with fewer repetitions.
- For advanced: Use heavier resistance or increase the number of repetitions for a more challenging workout.

28. Pool Noodle Bicycle: Add a twist to your leg workouts by using a pool noodle to perform bicycle exercises in the water.

- Step 1: Sit on a pool noodle, keeping it under your hips for support.
- Step 2: Engage your core and perform bicycle movements by pedaling your legs in the water.
- Step 3: Cycle for 2-3 minutes.

Muscle Groups: Pool noodle bicycle exercises work the core and leg muscles, including the quadriceps and hamstrings.

Modifications:

- For beginners: Use a larger or more buoyant noodle and start with a slower pace.
- For advanced: Use a narrower or thinner noodle or increase the speed of your leg cycling.

29. Water Treading with Medicine Ball: This challenging exercise combines water treading with the use of a medicine ball, improving your balance and coordination.

- Step 1: Stand in chest-deep water, holding a lightweight medicine ball in your hands.
- Step 2: Tread water while keeping the ball above the surface, using various movements to challenge your balance.

- Step 3: Tread for 2-3 minutes.

Muscle Groups: This exercise targets both upper and lower body muscles, focusing on arm strength and core stability.

Modifications:

- For beginners: Start with a lighter medicine ball or use a flotation device for support, and tread at a slower pace.
- For advanced: Use a heavier medicine ball or incorporate more complex movements and exercises.

30. Aqua Balance Exercises: We'll wrap up this chapter with a series of balance exercises that challenge your core and stability in a refreshing and serene aquatic environment.

- Step 1: Stand in chest-deep water, engaging your core to maintain balance.
- Step 2: Perform a series of balance exercises, such as standing on one leg,

lifting one leg to the side, or performing tree pose variations.

- Step 3: Focus on balance and stability for 2-3 minutes.

Muscle Groups: Aqua balance exercises target your core, leg muscles, and help improve overall balance and coordination.

Modifications:

- For beginners: Start with basic balance exercises and use a flotation device or noodle for support.
- For advanced: Challenge yourself with more complex balance poses and increase the duration of your balance practice.

With these 30 essential pool exercises, you have a comprehensive toolbox at your disposal, each movement carefully crafted to promote your physical fitness and overall well-being.

Whether your goal is to build strength, improve flexibility, enhance cardiovascular health, or simply indulge in the therapeutic embrace of water, these exercises offer a diverse range of options to cater to your unique needs.

Your fitness journey has only just begun, and these exercises are your trusty companions as you explore the wondrous world of pool workouts.

So, gear up in your swimwear, jump into the pool, and let's begin our journey of transforming your health and fitness through these 30 essential pool exercises for beginners.

Chapter four: Planning a Pool Workout

We've explored the tranquil waters of pool workouts, dipped our toes into the pool of benefits, and made our first steps toward a healthier, more active lifestyle in the prior chapters.

Now it's time to go deeper - to put on our swim caps and goggles and dive headfirst into the heart of your pool fitness journey.

This chapter is all about customization, the secret sauce that turns a workout into a transforming fitness experience. Welcome to the realm of designing a pool exercise plan, a blueprint customized to your own requirements, interests, and goals.

Why a Customized Pool Workout Plan Is Important

Consider a workout program that is as unique as you are. One that not only focuses on your personal goals but also values your uniqueness. That is exactly what a tailored pool exercise regimen provides. It's more than simply a set of exercises; it's a path that matches your goals and enhances your fitness journey.

Here's why it's important:

1. Increasing Outcomes: A tailored exercise plan guarantees that you are working towards the goals that are most important to you, whether they be muscle gain, flexibility improvement, or weight loss.

By focusing on your specific goals, you will see faster and more fulfilling outcomes.

2. Increased Pleasure: Exercising becomes more pleasurable when your training plan coincides with your hobbies and preferences. Instead of viewing your time in the pool as a nuisance, you'll look forward to it.

3. Improved Consistency: A strategy that fits your lifestyle is simpler to keep to. It reduces your chances of slipping off the exercise wagon and assists you in developing long-term, healthy habits.

4. Reduced Plateau Risk: A well-structured training regimen guarantees that you are always challenging your body. This keeps your development steady and minimizes plateaus.

5. Adherence and Safety: A tailored strategy takes into account your fitness level as well as any limits you may have, reducing the chance of injury and ensuring you can stick to your program.

Creating Your Own Pool Workout Routine

The formulation of a pool training plan is at the heart of the process. This chapter will teach you how to create a plan that works with your objectives, schedule, and physical ability.

We'll go over the following crucial points:

1. Goal Setting: Start by outlining your fitness objectives. What do you hope to accomplish with pool exercises? Clarifying your goals, whether it's better endurance, muscular tone, or relaxation, is the first step toward a successful strategy.

2. Assessing Your Fitness Level: Determine your present level of fitness. This evaluation aids in tailoring your strategy to your existing skills, ensuring that it is both challenging and doable.

3. Selecting the Appropriate Exercises: We'll go over some of the excellent exercises given earlier in the eBook, and you'll choose the ones that are most appropriate for your goals.

4. Planning Your Workouts: Discover how to plan your pool workouts, including warm-ups, primary exercises, and cool-downs. Find the ideal blend of aerobic, strength, and flexibility training.

5. Making a regimen: Learn how to make a fitness regimen that fits into your everyday routine. We'll look into weekly, biweekly, and monthly programs.

6. Tracking Your development: Recognize the significance of tracking your development and how to do so successfully. This crucial phase allows you to stay motivated and adjust your approach as needed.

7. Inspirational Plans: Throughout this chapter, you'll find sample exercise programs for a variety of goals, fitness levels, and schedules. These ideas are intended to serve as inspiration and templates that you may modify to meet your own requirements.

Creating a tailored pool exercise regimen is a trip inside a journey. It's an exciting undertaking that combines your goals with the fluid realm of water-based exercise.

This chapter gives you the skills and knowledge you need to create a strategy that guarantees your pool workout experience is not only productive but also genuinely pleasurable.

Are you ready to enter into the realm of customised pool training plans? Let's get started, creating a fitness journey that is uniquely yours, and enjoy the tremendous change that lies ahead.

Sample exercise regimens for beginners, moderate, and expert levels

When starting any fitness journey, it's critical to establish a plan that takes into account your present fitness level as well as your long-term goals. Pool exercises are no exception.

In this chapter, we'll look at some sample exercise regimens for beginners, intermediate enthusiasts, and experienced persons.

Each plan is painstakingly designed to harness the wonderful power of water, gently pushing your boundaries while respecting your body's particular demands.

1. Beginner's Workout Plan:

Getting Started in Fitness

Week 1 - 2: Introduction to Pool Exercises

Day 1 - 3: Begin with water walking. Spend 20 minutes walking back and forth in chest-deep water. Maintain excellent posture and controlled movements.

Day 4 - 7: Introduce leg raises. Stand in shoulder-deep water, hanging onto the pool's edge, and complete two sets of ten leg lifts for each leg.

Week 3 & 4: Increasing Endurance

Days 1 - 4: Continue water walking for 30 minutes. Experiment with different walking techniques, such as forward, backward, and sideways.

Day 5 - 7: Incorporate flutter kicks. Hold on to the pool's edge and do two sets of 12-15 flutter kicks.

2. Intermediate Workout Plan

Progress with Purpose

Week 1 - 2: Improving the Routine

Days 1 - 4: Increase water walking time to 45 minutes. Experiment with hand paddles or water weights to create resistance.

Day 5 - 7: Include knee-to-chest stretches in your workout. Perform two sets of ten stretches for each leg.

Week 3 - 4: Intensifying the Challenge

Day 1 - 4: For 45 minutes, alternate between water walking and running. Every two minutes, alternate between walking and running.

Day 5 - 7: Incorporate aquatic lunges. Stand in waist-deep water and do two sets of 12-15 lunges on each leg.

3. Advanced Workout Plan

Pushing Boundaries in the Pool

Week 1 & 2: Increasing Intensity

Day 1 - 4: Begin with a 15-minute warm-up of water walking or jogging. Then, for 30 seconds, conduct high-intensity water sprints followed by a 30-second rest. Repeat this cycle ten times.

Day 5 - 7: Incorporate deep water running with a flotation belt. Run in place for 20 minutes with maximal effort.

Week 3 & 4: Fine-Tuning Your Fitness

Day 1 - 5: Combine water jogging with resistance exercises.

For 30 minutes, use water paddles and employ high-intensity interval training **(HIIT)** bursts.

Day 5 - 7: Submerged push-ups will test your core and strength. Perform three sets of 12-15 push-ups.

These example workout routines serve as a starting point for your adventure with pool workouts, although they are by no means definitive. The beauty of aquatic fitness is its versatility.

Adjust the intensity, duration, and workouts to your personal development and comfort level. The most essential thing is to listen to your body, maintain consistency, and be committed to your wellness path.

By following these training regimens, you will gradually gain strength, improve your cardiovascular fitness, and gain a sense of success from pushing yourself inside the calming embrace of the water.

Remember that everyone learns at their own rate, so whether you're a beginner, an intermediate enthusiast, or an accomplished swimmer, there's a place for you in the world of pool workouts. Dive in and take on the task!

Tips on creating Goals and Tracking Progress: Charting Your Course to Success

Setting goals and measuring your progress are vital components of any fitness journey, and pool activities are no different. In reality, they are the compass and map that will lead you on your aquatic trip, ensuring that you stay motivated, make steady progress, and finally arrive at your destination - a healthier, happier you.

The Importance of Goal Setting

Goals are more than just abstract fantasies; they are definite, concrete ideas of your intended conclusion. Setting clear and attainable goals for your pool fitness regimen is critical to your success. Here's how to make goal setting work for you:

1. Define Your "Why: Begin by determining why you want to do pool exercises. Is it to enhance your cardiovascular health, relieve joint discomfort, lose weight, or simply live a more active lifestyle? Identifying your underlying drive will offer your objectives depth and purpose.

2. Establish SMART Goals: SMART stands for Specific, Measurable, Achievable, Relevant, and Time-bound. Your objectives should be clear and explicit, have a mechanism to monitor progress, be reasonable, link to your motivation, and have a timeline for completion.

A **SMART** goal would be: "I will swim for 30 minutes five days a week to lose 10 pounds in three months."

3. Prioritize Your Objectives: While having a list of objectives is beneficial, not all objectives are made equal. Prioritize them depending on what is most essential to you. Focusing on a few major goals at a time will help minimize overload.

4. Break It Down: Break down bigger goals into smaller, more achievable steps. If swimming a mile is your objective, start with lesser lengths and progressively work your way up. This method makes the journey more approachable and less intimidating.

Monitoring Progress

Setting goals is the initial step, but keeping track of your progress is what keeps you on track.

It acts as a source of inspiration, a means of making changes, and a means of celebrating your accomplishments.

Here's how to keep track of your progress:

1. Maintain a Workout notebook: Keep a notebook in which you document your exercises, including the type of exercise, duration, distance, and repetitions. This allows you to examine how far you've come and detect patterns in your development.

2. Apply Technology: Many fitness applications and wearable gadgets may assist you in tracking your exercises, including information such as distance, duration, calories burnt, and more. These tools make it simple to track your progress.

3. Take photographs and measurements: Visual signals may be extremely effective motivators. When you begin your trip, take "before" images and measurements and compare them to your present state at regular intervals. The visual changes will most likely surprise you.

4. Recognize Achievements: Recognize your development and appreciate your accomplishments, large and little. Reward yourself for reaching milestones and use these prizes to motivate you to achieve future objectives.

5. Regular Evaluations: Reevaluate your objectives on a regular basis. Are they still applicable? Do they need to be adjusted? Your objectives may change as you advance to match your evolving requirements and desires.

6. Stay Accountable: Discuss your objectives with a friend, gym companion, or a supportive community. Having people hold you accountable for your actions may be a tremendous incentive.

Remember that goals and progress monitoring are about more than simply getting to the finish line; they are also about the trip itself.

The daily dedication to your objectives, the sense of accomplishment as you cross off milestones, and the continuous quest of development are all essential components of your pool fitness experience.

Setting specific goals and evaluating your progress turns a passive fitness routine into an active and joyful journey.

Your goals serve as a compass, and progress monitoring serves as a road map to success, ensuring that your pool fitness trip is not only productive but also genuinely rewarding.

Set your goals, go on this journey, and enjoy the transformational power of pool workouts.

Your journey to better health and fitness begins right now.

Chapter Five: Motivation with Pool Exercises

When embarking on a fitness journey, motivation serves as your compass, directing you toward your objectives. However, motivation can be difficult to find, especially as the novelty of your fitness program wears off. This chapter is dedicated to keeping you motivated and excited about your pool workout adventure.

In the pages that follow, we'll look at tactics and insights to maintain your dedication to pool exercises steadfast, so you not only start strong but end strong.

Here you'll learn how to persevere, stay inspired, and cultivate a true enthusiasm for your aquatic exercises.

1. Setting Specific Goals: Motivation begins with a purpose. Define your fitness goals, both short and long term. Do you want to reduce weight, tone your muscles, enhance your cardiovascular health, or simply enjoy moving about in water? You'll have a clear picture of what you're working toward if you create specified, measurable, attainable, relevant, and time-bound (SMART) objectives.

2. Monitoring Your Progress:

Visualizing your accomplishments may be an effective motivator. Consider maintaining a workout log or utilizing a fitness app to track your progress and performance. Celebrate your successes, whether little or large, since they represent progress on your quest.

3. The Importance of Consistency:

The cornerstone of any exercise routine's success is consistency. Make an exercise regimen that you can reasonably stick to.

Your dedication will eventually turn into a habit, making exercise a natural part of your daily routine.

4. Experiment:

Variety is the spice of life, and it's equally important in your workout regimen. Pool exercises provide a plethora of alternatives. Change up your routines, attempt new exercises, and even test out new aquatic equipment. This keeps your motivation strong and minimizes boredom.

5 Motivational Enhancers:

Investigate many strategies for increasing your motivation. Music can be a strong motivator; make a playlist of your favorite songs to listen to while working out in the pool. For social support, you may also participate in friendly competitions with your training pals or attend water fitness courses.

6. Visualizing Success: Use your mind's power to visualize your desired outcomes. Visualize yourself reaching your fitness objectives. This mental rehearsal can strengthen your resolve and increase your self-esteem.

7. Look for Inspiration:

Inspiration may come from a variety of sources. Read success stories from people who have used pool activities to attain their fitness goals. Participate in online fitness forums and learn from the experiences of others.

8. Mark Milestones:

Don't forget to acknowledge your achievements. Reward yourself for reaching milestones with a treat, a soothing spa day, or any other sort of self-care that appeals to you.

9. Personal Affirmations:

Make up your own motivating affirmations to remind yourself of your potential, power, and perseverance. To keep your spirits up during your exercises, repeat these affirmations.

10. Monitor Your Emotional Health:

Take note of how pool workouts effect your mood and general well-being. Many people report less stress and more mental clarity following aquatic exercises, which may be encouraging.

Remember that motivation might fluctuate, which is completely natural. What's important is to devise ways for reigniting your enthusiasm when it wanes.

This chapter gives you the tools you need to achieve precisely that. Staying motivated and inspired on your pool workout adventure will allow you to continue reaping the numerous benefits that this unique kind of fitness provides.

Keep these encouraging methods handy as we move on. We're going to get into the core of pool exercises, looking at a variety of regimens that will stimulate your interest and keep your excitement strong.

Your fitness journey is a marathon, not a sprint, and you can complete it with vim and vitality if you have the correct motivation.

Let's continue our aquatic trip and learn how to take your pool fitness to new heights.

Strategies for Overcoming Common Obstacles in Pool Exercise:

Pool exercises may indeed be a transformative fitness option, but like any endeavor, they come with their unique set of challenges.

As you delve deeper into the world of aqua fitness, you might encounter some common obstacles. Fear not, for within this chapter, we'll equip you with effective strategies to conquer these hurdles and emerge from the waters stronger, more resilient, and ready to excel in your pool exercise routine.

1. Time Management difficulty:

Obstacle: Finding time for exercise can be a daunting challenge in our hectic lives. The pool may be accessible, but squeezing in a workout amidst your daily responsibilities may seem impossible.

Strategy: Prioritizing your health is the first step. Assess your daily schedule and identify windows of opportunity. Set realistic goals and allocate specific time slots for your pool exercises.

Consider it a non-negotiable appointment with yourself, just like any other commitment.

2. Motivation Blues:

Obstacle: Staying motivated can be difficult, especially when the initial enthusiasm begins to wane, and the novelty of pool exercises wears off.

Strategy: Keep your motivation aflame by setting clear, achievable goals. Break down your fitness journey into manageable milestones, and celebrate each accomplishment. Consider enlisting a workout buddy or joining a class to stay accountable and foster camaraderie. Music can also be a powerful motivator – create a pool exercise playlist to keep you moving.

3. Perceived Monotony:

Obstacle: Some beginners may perceive pool exercises as monotonous, fearing they might quickly grow tired of the same routines.

Strategy: Inject variety into your workouts. Explore different exercises, add new challenges, and mix up your routine to keep things fresh.

Try water aerobics classes or experiment with aquatic equipment like resistance bands and pool noodles to diversify your experience.

4. Self-Consciousness:

Obstacle: It's not uncommon to feel self-conscious when you start pool exercises. The thought of being seen in a swimsuit or not knowing the routines can be intimidating.

Strategy: Remember that everyone starts somewhere, and the pool is a judgment-free zone. Choose a time to exercise when the pool is less crowded, allowing you to build your confidence gradually.

Consider wearing a comfortable swimsuit that makes you feel confident and focus on your progress, not on what others may think.

5. Plateaus and Frustration:

Obstacle: After initial progress, you may hit a plateau where it seems like you're not improving or achieving your fitness goals.

Strategy: Plateaus are a natural part of any fitness journey. To overcome them, try adjusting your routines, increasing intensity, or setting new goals. Regularly challenge yourself with different exercises and keep a record of your workouts to track your progress and recognize improvements.

6. Weather and Seasonal Limitations:

Obstacle: Outdoor pool access may be restricted during certain seasons, making it challenging to maintain your pool exercise routine.

Strategy: Investigate indoor pool options, consider alternative activities during off-seasons, or adapt your routine for land-based workouts. Remember that setbacks due to weather or seasonal changes are temporary, and maintaining a consistent fitness regimen remains the ultimate goal.

7. Fear of Water:

Obstacle: Some beginners may be uneasy or fearful of water, which can hinder their participation in pool exercises.

Strategy: Start with water activities that don't involve submersion, such as water walking or exercises in shallower areas. Gradually build confidence and overcome your fears by taking small, consistent steps. If necessary, consider seeking guidance from a professional swimming instructor.

8. Navigating Health Challenges:

Obstacle: Health issues, such as injuries or medical conditions, may pose unique challenges for pool exercises.

Strategy: Consult with a healthcare professional to determine what exercises are safe and beneficial for your specific condition. Many pool exercises are low-impact and can be adapted to accommodate various health challenges, so your healthcare provider can help tailor a plan suitable for your needs.

By implementing these strategies, you'll be better equipped to navigate and overcome the common obstacles that may arise in your pool exercise journey.

Remember, every challenge is an opportunity for growth, and the path to fitness is a dynamic one. Dive in with determination, and with the right strategies in place, you'll ride the waves of success to a healthier, happier you.

Chapter Six: Nutrition diet and Hydration Strategy

While pool workouts provide a novel approach to training, it's critical to remember that food and hydration are critical to your overall performance. What you eat and drink has a significant impact on your energy levels, endurance, and the efficacy of your exercises. As a result, we've dedicated this part to developing a meal plan and hydration strategy just for pool exercisers, assuring you have the nutrition and sustenance you need to make the most of your aquatic undertakings.

The ABCs of Eating Right

Before we get into the specifics of a meal plan, let's go over some fundamental ideas that can guide your food choices as a pool exerciser.

1. Balanced Nutrients: A well-balanced diet is critical. Incorporate carbs, proteins, healthy fats, vitamins, and minerals into your diet. These nutrients give your body with the fuel and support it requires for prolonged workout and recuperation.

2. Time Is Everything: When you eat is just as important as what you consume. Consuming a balanced lunch or snack approximately 1-2 hours before your pool workout session can offer the essential energy without causing discomfort in the water.

3. Post-Workout Nutrition: Following your pool session, it's critical to have a meal or snack that restores the nutrients you've lost during exercise. This aids in muscle repair and reduces post-workout weariness.

Example Meal Plan for Pool Exercisers

Breakfast:

- Greek yogurt with fresh berries and a drizzle of honey
- Whole-grain toast with almond butter
- A glass of water or herbal tea

Lunch:

- Grilled chicken breast or tofu with a big serving of mixed veggies
- Quinoa or brown rice - A side salad with a little vinaigrette dressing
- A glass of lemon-flavored water

Snack:

- A banana or a handful of mixed almonds
- A glass of water

Pre-Workout Snack (1-2 hours before exercise):

- A modest portion of oats or a whole-grain cereal bar
- A glass of water

Post-Workout Meal or Snack:

- A smoothie blended with your choice of protein powder, spinach, banana, and almond milk.
- Whole-grain crackers with hummus
- A glass of water

Dinner:

- Grilled salmon or a plant-based protein source such as lentils
- Steamed broccoli or other green vegetables
- Quinoa or whole-grain pasta
- A glass of water or herbal tea

Pool Hydration Strategies:

Proper hydration is critical to pool performance. Even if you don't see yourself sweating, the combination of exertion and the aquatic environment can cause increased perspiration and fluid loss.

Dehydration may affect your physical ability as well as offer health dangers, therefore it's critical to maintain a constant hydration regimen.

Pre-Hydration: Begin your day with a glass of water and stay hydrated throughout the day. Drink water steadily rather than in excessive quantities soon before your pool practice. Dehydration can begin before you feel thirsty, so it's critical to start your workout well-hydrated.

During Exercise: Hydration is crucial for pool activities, but bear in mind that you may not feel as thirsty in the water.

Drink water between sets or workouts to keep hydrated. Aim for 7-10 ounces of water per 10-20 minutes of activity.

Post-Exercise Hydration: Restore fluids lost during exertion after your workout. Rehydrating with water, coconut water, or an electrolyte-containing sports drink might be useful.

Final Thoughts

Your meal plan and hydration approach should be adaptive to your unique tastes and dietary constraints.

The objective is to sufficiently fuel your body before and after pool exercises, as well as to keep hydrated throughout your workout.

By including a balanced diet plan and sufficient hydration into your training program, you are not only enhancing your performance in the water but also boosting your entire health and well-being.

The combination of healthy meals and adequate hydration is your secret weapon for getting the most of your pool activities and ensuring that each splash in the pool puts you closer to your fitness objectives.

Stay nourished, stay refreshed, and keep creating waves on your aquatic path to health and vitality.

Chapter Seven: Recovery and Self-Care

In the hustle and bustle of contemporary life, we frequently overlook the value of recuperation and self-care in our exercise regimens.

We put our body through strenuous activities and then go on to the next activity without taking the time to allow our muscles recuperate and our thoughts relax.

In this chapter, we'll highlight the importance of post-workout recovery and self-care in the realm of pool workouts.

The Art of Recovery

1. Recognizing Recovery: Recovery is more than just the time you spend relaxing after a workout; it's an important stage in your fitness journey. During this period, your body restores and strengthens itself, allowing you to proceed successfully.

We'll look at the science of recuperation and how it affects muscle growth and general health.

2. Hydration and Nutrition: Proper post-workout nutrition is critical for recovery. Learn what to eat and drink after pool activities to refill your energy and help your body's natural healing processes.

3. Foam rolling and stretching: Investigate the advantages of foam rolling and stretching for muscular tightness and flexibility.

We'll present hands-on demonstrations and strategies that you may include into your post-workout routine.

4. Sleep and Stress Management: Sleep is the body's natural recuperation process.

Learn how to improve your sleep habits and stress management practices to give your body the greatest opportunity to recover and replenish.

Self-Care for Holistic Well-Being

5. The Mind-Body Connection: Recognize the significant link between your mental and physical wellness. We'll go over several mindfulness techniques that can help you improve your self-care routine.

6. Relaxation Techniques: Learn the art of relaxation via techniques such as meditation, deep breathing, and gradual muscle relaxation. These approaches will assist you in finding peace and tranquillity in your hectic life.

7. Damage Prevention: Pool workouts are recognized for their low-impact nature, which reduces the chance of damage.

Nonetheless, we'll provide advice on how to avoid common pool accidents and practice pool safety.

8. Self-Care Rituals: Self-care is a lifestyle that includes your everyday decisions, not only what happens after a workout. We'll walk you through the process of developing self-care rituals, from morning routines to nighttime wind-downs.

Developing a Self–Care Routine

9. Self-Care in Action: We'll share real-life tales of people who have made self-care and recovery an important part of their fitness journey. Their experiences will motivate you to do the same.

10. Establishing a Support System: A good support system may have a big influence on your self-care journey. Learn how to build connections and resources that promote your well-being.

In this chapter, we'll look at the art of healing and self-care in the context of pool workouts. You'll realize that recuperation isn't only about sitting motionless, but also about engaging in activities and routines that encourage healing and growth.

Self-care is a comprehensive approach to well-being that focuses on your physical, mental, and emotional health, and we'll help you develop a self-care lifestyle that compliments your fitness journey.

So, let's dig into the art of recovery and self-care and embrace a lifestyle that not only encourages fitness but also supports your body, mind, and soul.

Conclusion: Begin Living a Wellness Life

As we complete our examination of pool workouts for beginners, it's time to reflect on the fantastic experience we've shared.

We've dabbled in the revitalizing world of aquatic exercise, found the numerous advantages that lie inside the tranquil waters of a pool, and armed ourselves with the information, motivation, and tools to embark on a transforming path toward health and well-being.

Recap the Key Takeaways

We've discussed the several advantages of pool exercises throughout this eBook, from low-impact, joint-friendly workouts to the stress-relieving and varied character of these aquatic routines. We've examined 30 key pool workouts, each of which is intended to shape your body and revive your mind.

We've looked at how to make personalized training regimens that are tailored to your fitness level and goals. We understand the importance of nutrition, hydration, and self-care in improving the pool workout experience.

We've hailed the possibility of unlimited advancement and lifelong fitness. Above all, we've laid the groundwork for you to experience the joys of living an active, healthy, and holistic lifestyle.

Key Takeaways from this eBook

1. Everyone can benefit from pool exercises: Pool workouts are a gentle yet powerful approach to keep active and preserve your health, regardless of your age, fitness level, or physical condition.

2. Physical and Mental Health: Pool workouts offer mental clarity, stress reduction, and a sense of peace that is frequently difficult to achieve elsewhere.

3. Variability and Pleasure: The pool is your blank canvas, where you may create a workout plan according to your interests and goals. Pool exercises are all about having fun.

4. Nutrition and Hydration Are Important: What you eat and drink is just as important as your training regimen. We've spoken about how appropriate diet and hydration may boost your performance.

5. Consistency is Essential: In any fitness endeavor, staying motivated and consistent is a huge obstacle. We've given tips for staying on track and excited about your success.

Encourage Pool Exercise Inception

As we get to the end of our voyage, there is no better time than now to begin your pool workout experience. The pool is your retreat, where wellness meets water where health and happiness are inextricably linked.

It's not a distant fantasy, but a realistic and approachable reality just waiting for you to take the leap.

Here's your invitation to adopt a way of life that prioritizes your well-being, blends fun with exercise, and goes beyond the limitations of standard fitness programs.

It's an open invitation to investigate the tremendous, transformational potential of pool workouts, and we urge you to accept it enthusiastically.

So put on your swimwear, collect your drive, and dive into the sea with zeal. Your fitness adventure in the realm of pool workouts for beginners begins right now.

The advantages, delight, and sense of well-being you've read about are more than just words on a page; they're experiences waiting for you beneath the water's surface.

Remember that each stroke, movement, and minute in the water pushes you closer to being a healthier, happier, and more vibrant version of yourself.

Each day of exercise will make you feel a bit stronger, more balanced, and full of energy. And when the water surrounds you, not just your body but also your attitude on life changes.

So, let's end with a splash, a leap, and a pledge to a better, more active lifestyle. Your journey begins here, and your objective is a life filled with the energy of water and the wealth of health. Dive in, embrace the realm of basic pool workouts, and let the journey begin.

Thank you for reading

Printed in Great Britain
by Amazon

42549842R00076